GAPS DIET

FOR NOVICES

Enriched Recipes, Foods, Meal Plan & Procedures That Focuses On Digestive Health, Gut Brain Relationship, Dealing With Depression, Anxiety And More

DR. MATEO GABRIEL

DISCLAIMER

The information in this book is only meant to be used for general reading. In any way, the author and publisher do not promise or represent that the information in this work is full, correct, reliable, appropriate, or available. This includes any warranties that are expressed or implied. Because of this, you should only rely on this material at your own risk.

This book is not meant to replace professional help. If you have any questions about a subject, you should always get help from a qualified expert. The author and distributor of this book are not responsible for how the information in it is used or abused.

The author's thoughts and feelings are shown in this book. They do not necessarily represent the official policy or stance of any other person, group, employer, or business.

Any third-party material that you can get to through this book is not endorsed or backed by the author or publisher.

The information in this book is correct at the time it was published, after all possible checks. However, the author and distributor are not responsible for any loss, damage, or inconvenience that may be caused by mistakes or omissions.

TABLE OF CONTENTS

CHAPTER ONE

INTRODUCTION TO GAPS DIET

AN OUTLINE OF THE GAPS DIET

A diet plan called the Gut and Psychology Syndrome diet (GAPS diet) was made to look at the link between gut health and overall health. The GAPS Diet was created by neurologist and nutritionist Dr. Natasha Campbell-McBride. It is based on the idea that a weakened digestive system may be a factor in several physical and mental health conditions. The regimen addresses everything from neurological and psychological illnesses to digestive issues, with the ultimate goal of sealing and healing the gut lining.

The fundamental tenet of the GAPS Diet is that a variety of health issues can arise from an unbalanced gut microbiome, which is defined as an excess of pathogenic bacteria and a shortage of helpful bacteria. The regimen calls for avoiding some processed meals, carbohydrates, and sweets and emphasizing the eating of nutrient-dense, whole foods. The GAPS Diet attempts to assist in the restoration of healthy gut flora in this way since it is thought to be essential for achieving the best possible physical and mental health.

THE VALUE OF DIGESTIVE HEALTH

Beyond the particular procedure, the GAPS Diet's core idea of gut health is significant. The stomach, sometimes called the "second brain," is essential to the body's general operation. Trillions of bacteria called the gut microbiota live there and have an impact on the immune system, nutritional absorption, and digestion. The gut-brain axis has also received attention from recent studies, which show that the stomach and the central nervous system communicate in both directions and can affect mood, thought processes, and even behavior.

HISTORICAL CONTEXT

Gaining knowledge about the GAPS Diet's past might help you better understand how it has developed and changed over time. The regimen was developed by Dr. Natasha Campbell-McBride, drawing from her clinical background in treating patients with neurological and psychosocial conditions, especially children. She discovered a similarity among many of her patients—a damaged state of gut health—by utilizing her medical training and observations. The GAPS Diet was created as a comprehensive strategy to treat the underlying problems causing a variety of health concerns as a result of this discovery.

The scientific and medical societies' evolving understanding of the gut-brain connection is intricately linked to the historical background of the GAPS Diet. The GAPS Diet is a groundbreaking dietary plan that highlights the role of diet in promoting healthy gut microbiota and, therefore, general health, as research continues to unearth the complex relationships between gut health and many facets of well-being.

CHAPTER TWO

KNOWLEDGE OF THE GUT-BRAIN RELATIONSHIP

THE BRAIN-GUT AXIS

The gastrointestinal tract and the brain are connected by a bidirectional communication mechanism known as the Gut-Brain Axis (GBA). This complex network includes the enteric nervous system (ENS), the central nervous system (CNS), and the large population of gut-dwelling bacteria, or gut microbiota. These components communicate with each other via a variety of signaling channels, such as hormonal, immunological, and neurological ones.

This intricate interaction is essential for controlling not only the digestive system but also the brain and emotions.

GUT HEALTH'S EFFECT ON MENTAL HEALTH

Recent years have seen a notable increase in the amount of research focused on the relationship between gut health and mental health. Growing research indicates that dysbiosis, or abnormalities in the makeup of the gut microbiota, can have a significant impact on mood, stress response, and cognitive performance. Numerous bioactive substances, including neurotransmitters and short-chain fatty acids, that might affect brain activity and communication are produced by the gut bacteria. Furthermore, because the stomach plays a major role in the immune system, disruptions in gut health have been connected to inflammatory diseases that may exacerbate mental health issues.

Studies have shown links between disorders such as anxiety, depression, and even neurodegenerative diseases and changes in the gut flora. Beneficial bacteria known as probiotics have been studied for their potential to improve mental health by reestablishing a balanced gut flora.

Diet, exercise, and sleep patterns are important lifestyle factors that also have a significant impact on gut health and, by extension, mental health outcomes. Targeting and comprehending the gut-brain axis may provide novel therapeutic approaches for the treatment of mental health conditions.

SCIENCE BEHIND THE GAPS DIET

The foundation of the Gut and Psychology Syndrome (GAPS) diet is the idea that several physical and mental health problems can be linked to an unhealthy gut. Dr. Natasha Campbell-McBride created the diet plan, based on her theory that eating particular foods can worsen gut dysbiosis and cause leaky gut and systemic inflammation.

The GAPS diet promotes the ingestion of nutrient-dense, easily digestible foods while emphasizing the elimination of specific food groups, such as grains, processed foods, and sweets.

The GAPS diet's focus on regaining gut health through nutrition for the gut lining and beneficial bacteria populations forms its scientific foundation. The goal of the diet is to balance the gut bacteria, encourage the healing of the gut lining, and lessen inflammation. The scientific agreement regarding the GAPS diet's effectiveness for certain ailments is still developing, even though some people claim benefits for a variety of health issues after implementing it.

More thorough scientific research, according to critics, is necessary to substantiate the diet's promises and comprehend its long-term impacts on mental and intestinal health.

CHAPTER THREE

CONDITIONS GAPS DIET ADDRESSES

AUTISM SPECTRUM DISORDERS

Due to its possible effects on people with ASD, the GAPS (Gut and Psychology Syndrome) diet has drawn interest. The GAPS diet's proponents think there's a link between neurological disorders like ASD and gut health. The diet's main goals are to repair the gut lining and encourage the development of healthy bacteria in the digestive tract. The GAPS diet is expected to have a positive impact on ASD symptoms by treating inflammation and gut dysbiosis. While studies on this particular component are still in their infancy, anecdotal evidence and personal success stories indicate that some people who follow the GAPS protocol report improvements in their behavior, communication, and social interactions.

ADHD: People who suffer from Attention Deficit Hyperactivity Disorder (ADHD) frequently struggle with impulsivity, hyperactivity, and attention span issues. According to the GAPS diet, abnormalities in the gut flora may be a factor in neurological problems that impact behavior and cognitive abilities. The GAPS diet attempts to treat underlying gut problems that may have an impact on brain function by emphasizing a nutrient-dense, gut-healing approach. Following the GAPS treatment, some people have reported increases in their ability to focus, pay attention, and maintain behavioral control. It is important to remember that there is currently little scientific proof that the GAPS diet is effective for treating ADHD, and more studies are required to confirm the diet's effectiveness as a therapeutic strategy.

DEPRESSION AND ANXIETY

A key component of the GAPS diet is the relationship between gut health and mental health. Inflammation, impaired gut barrier function, and abnormalities in the gut flora are frequently associated with depression and anxiety. The GAPS diet places a strong emphasis on eating wholesome, easily digested foods to promote gut healing and the development of good bacteria. Supporters of the GAPS protocol contend that improving gut health can have a beneficial impact on neurotransmitter synthesis and lower systemic inflammation, which may lessen anxiety and depressive symptoms. These assertions are supported by some anecdotal data, but scientific study on the precise effects of the GAPS diet on mental health disorders is still in its infancy.

AUTOIMMUNE DISORDERS

The GAPS diet targets the gut, which is the primary source of many health problems, to treat autoimmune disorders. The GAPS protocol's proponents contend that autoimmune illnesses can arise as a result of damaged gut lining. By avoiding some foods that may cause immunological reactions and encouraging the consumption of nutrient-dense, therapeutic foods, the diet seeks to improve gut health, lower inflammation, and rebalance the immune system. Although some people with autoimmune disorders say that the GAPS diet helps with their symptoms, it is important to treat these claims cautiously because there isn't any solid scientific data to support the GAPS diet's efficacy for autoimmune conditions.

DIGESTIVE PROBLEMS

The main goal of the GAPS diet is to promote gut healing to treat a range of digestive problems. Increased intestinal permeability and abnormalities in the gut microbiota are thought to play a role in the development of conditions like leaky gut syndrome, irritable bowel syndrome (IBS), and inflammatory bowel disorders (IBD). To stimulate gut repair, the GAPS protocol encourages the use of bone broths, fermented foods, and nutrient-dense foods while advocating the elimination of other foods that may exacerbate these problems. Following the GAPS diet, some people with digestive issues report feeling better and having fewer symptoms. The scientific community does, however, stress the necessity for additional studies to determine the diet's effectiveness and comprehend its effects on different digestive disorders.

CHAPTER FOUR

BEGINNING TO USE GAPS

GETTING READY EMOTIONALLY AND MENTALLY

One of the most important things before starting the Gut and Psychology Syndrome (GAPS) diet is to psychologically and emotionally prepare. A new diet can be difficult to adjust to, so it's important to go into it with an optimistic outlook and a dedication to bettering your general health. Learning the fundamentals of the GAPS diet and its possible effects on mental and emotional well-being is advantageous. People can more successfully manage the early phases of the diet by setting attainable goals and realistic expectations.

CONSULTATION WITH MEDICAL EXPERTS

Before beginning the GAPS diet, it is essential to speak with medical authorities, especially if you are taking medication or have pre-existing health conditions. Dietitians, nutritionists, and practitioners of functional medicine are examples of healthcare specialists who can offer tailored guidance based on a patient's unique health requirements. This partnership guarantees that the dietary adjustments are safe and in line with overall health objectives.

Speaking with a healthcare expert can also help identify possible obstacles and create a tailored plan to address specific health issues.

TOOLS AND KITCHEN PREPARATION

Having the right tools and kitchen prep is essential to following the GAPS diet. It is necessary to get rid of processed foods, sugar, and other non-compliant things to make a kitchen GAPS-friendly. Having a well-stocked kitchen with appliances like a blender, fermenting jars, and a high-quality stockpot makes cooking healthful and digestible meals easier. Setting up the kitchen to use only GAPS-compatible ingredients and getting rid of anything that isn't compliant contributes to a welcoming atmosphere for sticking to the diet plan.

KEEP GAPS-FRIENDLY INGREDIENTS ON HAND

Keeping GAPS-friendly foods on hand is essential to properly executing the diet. Give top priority to complete, high-nutrient foods like veggies, fermented dairy products, organic meats, and bone broth. Obtaining premium, ideally organic, products is crucial for maximizing nutritional intake and reducing exposure to potentially hazardous contaminants.

CHAPTER FIVE

THE INTRODUCTION DIET OF GAPS

PHASES AND STAGES

A therapy program called the GAPS (Gut and Psychology Syndrome) Introduction Diet aims to heal and address gut-related disorders, emphasizing the complex relationship between the gut and a range of neurological and psychological conditions. The diet is divided into multiple phases and stages, each of which is thoughtfully designed to progressively add and remove particular items. These phases seek to support the repair of the intestinal lining, restore equilibrium to the gut flora, and reduce symptoms related to a range of illnesses.

To give the digestive system a break, the first phases of the GAPS Introduction Diet concentrate on meals that are high in nutrients and easily digested. First-stage foods include fermented meals high in probiotics, well-cooked vegetables, and homemade broths made with meat and vegetables. More foods like eggs, and ghee, and progressively more complex carbs like fruits and honey are added as people advance through the phases. Reintroducing a range of foods gradually is the aim, and all the while, the body's reaction is being closely observed to detect any possible sensitivities or responses.

FOODS TO TAKE AND LEAVE OUT

During the GAPS Introduction Diet, some foods are strictly prohibited while others are recommended. The diet promotes the consumption of foods high in nutrients and low in digestion, such as fermented vegetables, bone broths, and dairy products with lots of probiotics, such as homemade yogurt. These meals are thought to support microbial balance and intestinal healing. In contrast, processed meals, sweets, grains, and starchy vegetables are usually avoided in the early phases to lighten the load on the digestive tract and limit any possible irritations.

EXAMPLES OF MENUS

Making nutritious and well-balanced meal plans is crucial to the GAPS Introduction Diet's success. Sample menus frequently feature fermented foods like sauerkraut, well-cooked vegetables, and soups prepared from scratch using bone broth. Meal diversity increases as people move through the phases, incorporating more proteins, good fats, and particular types of carbs. Meal plans should be customized to each person's tastes and dietary restrictions while following the stage-specific recommendations.

HANDLING THE SYMPTOMS OF DETOX

Managing detox symptoms is an essential part of the GAPS Introduction Diet since the healing process may cause the body to shift significantly. Fatigue, headaches, and stomach discomfort are some of the symptoms of detoxification. It's advised to get enough sleep, drink enough of water, and incorporate detoxifying activities like Epsom salt baths or skin brushing. Those who are familiar with the GAPS protocol and constantly monitor their symptoms can effectively manage the symptoms of detoxification and make necessary dietary adjustments.

The secret to executing the GAPS Introduction Diet successfully is to be patient and move slowly through the stages, letting the body repair and adjust at its rate.

CHAPTER SIX

GAPS WHOLE FOOD

MAKING THE SWITCH FROM INTRODUCTION TO COMPLETE DIET

A critical stage in the Gut and Psychology Syndrome (GAPS) therapy, which aims to repair and seal the gut lining while regaining optimal gut function, is the switch from the Introduction Diet to the Full GAPS Diet. By introducing foods that are readily digested and giving the stomach time to gradually adjust, the Introduction Diet acts as a preliminary phase. People proceed toward the Full GAPS Diet, which broadens the list of permissible foods. This change is predicated on the idea that the introduction phase caused the gut to recover significantly, strengthening it and increasing its capacity to process a wider variety of meals.

GAPS FOODS, BOTH LEGAL AND ILLEGAL

Foods are divided into two primary categories within the framework of the GAPS protocol: legal and illegal. Foods classified as legal are those that are thought to promote intestinal healing and are safe to eat. These usually consist of foods that are high in nutrients and are simple to digest, like fermented veggies, homemade broths, organic meats, and healthy fats like olive and coconut oils. Illegal meals, on the other hand, are those that can impede healing and make intestinal problems worse. Processed foods, grains, refined sugars, and some dairy items are frequently included in this group.

MAKING GAPS MEALS THAT ARE BALANCED

On the GAPS diet, meal timing is crucial for giving the body the nutrients it needs and encouraging gut healing. Healthy fats, non-starchy veggies, and a source of high-quality protein are usually included in a well-rounded GAPS diet. Avocados, almonds, seeds, and cold-pressed oils are good sources of healthful fats, while grass-fed meats, poultry, fish, and eggs are good sources of protein. Because of their high fiber content and nutritional profile, non-starchy veggies are recommended. This mixture guarantees a wide range of nutrients that aid in the healing process in addition to promoting general health.

PLANNING MEALS FOR VARIOUS STAGES

A crucial part of the GAPS protocol is meal planning, especially as participants move through the diet's phases. Meals on the Introduction Diet are purposefully restricted to foods that are simple to digest, like soups, broths, and boiled meats. Meal planning becomes more varied as people adopt the Full GAPS Diet, including a greater variety of foods while still avoiding certain triggers. During this phase, it is important to take individual tolerance, preferences, and nutritional demands into account. Making meal plans in advance guarantees that the body gets a balanced variety of nutrients for the best possible healing and gut restoration, as well as supporting adherence to the regimen.

CHAPTER SEVEN
MEAL IDEAS AND RECIPES
BREAKFAST

Often seen as the most significant meal of the day, breakfast gives you the energy you need to go through the morning. To maintain energy levels throughout the day, a well-balanced breakfast should contain a mix of carbohydrates, protein, and healthy fats. Popular traditional alternatives include whole-grain bread with avocado, yogurt with fruits, and porridge. Smoothie bowls, loaded with fruits, veggies, and seeds, are a light and healthy way to get started.

LUNCH

Lunch is a chance to replenish energy and keep your attention for the remainder of the day. Creating a meal that is both satiating and nourishing requires including a range of food types. A well-rounded alternative is a salad made up of a variety of vibrant veggies, lean meats like grilled chicken or tofu, and a hearty grain like brown rice or quinoa. For people who are often on the go, wraps or sandwiches stuffed with lean meats, vegetables, and a tasty spread offer a quick and portable meal option.

DINNER

Dinner is a time to relax and provide the body with a healthy, well-balanced meal. A satisfying and nourishing meal is made with a protein source—fish, poultry, or plant-based alternatives—a large portion of veggies, and a complex carbohydrate—sweet potatoes or whole-grain pasta. Your evening meals will taste better and be more fun if you experiment with different herbs and spices.

SNACKS

Eating a snack in between meals can help you stay energized and avoid overindulging in your main meals.

Selecting snacks that are high in nutrients is essential for promoting general health. A balanced balance of vitamins, minerals, and lipids can be found in fresh fruits, raw veggies with hummus, or a handful of mixed nuts. Protein, probiotics, and carbohydrates are all combined in a tasty and filling snack that is Greek yogurt with oats and honey drizzled over top.

DESSERTS

There are many methods to make sweet sweets using healthy ingredients, and desserts can be enjoyed as part of a balanced diet. Desserts including fruit, like baked apples or grilled peaches, naturally have sweetness without the need for extra sugar. When eaten in moderation, dark chocolate's antioxidant qualities can make it an indulgence guilt-free. Try experimenting with different sweeteners in baking recipes, such as honey or maple syrup, to give traditional desserts a healthy makeover.

DRINKS

Drinking enough water is important, and making the appropriate beverage choices can improve general health. While water is always the best option, herbal teas, and infused water can offer some variation without adding any extra sugar. When ingested in moderation, freshly squeezed juices provide an additional vitamin boost.

Smoothies are a convenient and hydrating way to add nutrients to your diet. They are produced with a combination of fruits, vegetables, and a protein source such as protein powder or yogurt. Reducing your use of sugar-filled sodas and choosing unsweetened substitutes can guarantee that the beverages you choose support your health objectives.

CHAPTER EIGHT

FRIENDLY FERMENTED FOODS FOR GAPS

THE SIGNIFICANCE OF FERMENTED MEALS

The GAPS (Gut and Psychology Syndrome) diet is heavily reliant on fermented foods, which have numerous advantages for gut health and general well-being. The capacity of fermented foods to support a diversified and well-balanced microbiota explains their significance in this dietary strategy. Beneficial microorganisms like bacteria and yeast aid in the fermentation process by breaking down the sugars and starches in food to produce lactic acid and other chemicals. These byproducts add probiotics that promote a healthy intestinal environment in addition to aiding in the food's preservation.

Fermented foods that are GAPS-friendly are important because they improve the absorption of nutrients and digestion. Certain food ingredients are predigested during the fermentation process, which facilitates the body's absorption of nutrients. This is especially crucial for GAPS dieters because their digestive systems are frequently impaired. Frequent consumption of fermented foods can support the development of a strong and resilient gut flora, which enhances general health.

METHODS FOR FERMENTING VEGETABLES

Fermented vegetable recipes are easy to make at home and quite satisfying. Start by choosing fresh, organic veggies like cucumbers, carrots, and cabbage. After chopping or slicing the veggies, toss them with sea salt and let it extract moisture. The next step is to make sure the vegetables are completely soaked in their juices by packing them snugly into a clean, airtight container. Depending on personal taste preferences, let the veggies ferment at room temperature for a predetermined amount of time, usually a few days to a few weeks. The outcome is a batch of nutritious and tasty fermented veggies that can be used in a variety of GAPS-friendly recipes.

DAIRY CULTURE ON THE GAPS DIET

Another important GAPS diet skill is cultivating dairy, which offers a source of probiotics and helpful enzymes. Dairy that is raw or organic is better since it has more good bacteria in it. Dairy must be cultured by adding a starter culture or using a tiny quantity of fermented dairy as a starter. After that, this combination is allowed to ferment at a regulated temperature until it thickens and takes on a tart taste.

The resulting cultured dairy products, which are rich in nutrients and can be ingested as part of the GAPS diet, include yogurt and kefir.

INCLUDING FERMENTED FOODS IN YOUR EVERYDAY MEALS

It takes imagination and a willingness to try new flavors and textures to incorporate fermented foods into regular GAPS diet meals. Vegetables that have undergone fermentation can be eaten as a side dish, mixed into salads, or even used in main meals. Dairy products with culture, such as kefir and yogurt, can be eaten on their own or as a foundation for sauces and smoothies.

People following the GAPS diet can achieve optimal gut health and enjoy a tasty, high-nutrient meal by varying the kinds of fermented foods they consume and combining them into different dishes.

CHAPTER NINE

SUPPORT FOR NUTRITION AND LIFESTYLE

STRESS MANAGEMENT

Stress negatively affects people's general well-being and is an unavoidable aspect of life. Managing stress well is essential to keeping up a healthy lifestyle. Numerous physical and mental health conditions, including anxiety disorders, compromised immune systems, and cardiovascular difficulties, can be brought on by prolonged stress. People can manage stress better by implementing stress-reduction strategies like deep breathing exercises, mindfulness meditation, and taking regular pauses. A more robust and balanced way of living can also result from partaking in enjoyable and soothing activities, such as hobbies or time spent in nature.

The importance of getting enough good sleep is essential for maintaining optimum health and well-being. Sleep is essential for several physiological functions, such as memory consolidation, immunological response, and cellular repair. Chronic sleep deprivation has been associated with an increased risk of developing heart disease, diabetes, and obesity. Promoting restorative sleep requires developing a regular sleep schedule, furnishing a cozy sleeping space, and adhering to excellent sleep hygiene. Not only does getting enough sleep improve physical health, but it also improves emotional control, cognitive performance, and general quality of life.

SUPPLEMENTS FOR THE GAPS DIET

The Gut and Psychology Syndrome (GAPS) diet is a dietary strategy intended to promote gut health and treat a range of illnesses, such as neurological and digestive diseases. Although whole foods are the main focus of the GAPS diet, several supplements are frequently suggested to enhance the nutritional aspects of the regimen.

Probiotics are essential for maintaining a healthy immune system, helping with digestion, and supporting gut flora. Supplements like zinc, vitamin D, and omega-3 fatty acids may also be added to correct nutritional shortages and promote general well-being. It's critical to customize supplement use based on unique requirements and seek the guidance of a healthcare provider for specific recommendations.

EXERCISE & PHYSICAL EXERCISE

Having a regular physical exercise schedule is essential to living a healthy lifestyle, as it provides numerous advantages for both mental and physical health. Improved physical strength and flexibility, weight control, and cardiovascular health are all benefits of exercise. Exercise has psychological advantages in addition to physical ones. It also lowers stress and improves mood and cognitive performance. Exercise can take many forms and intensities, from strength training and yoga to cardiovascular pursuits like running or cycling, depending on personal preferences and fitness levels. promotes general health and energy.

CHAPTER TEN
COMMON DIFFICULTIES
HANDLING PLATEAUS

In attempts to lose weight or improve fitness, plateaus can be discouraging and annoying. A frequent problem people encounter is the seeming stagnation of progress despite persistent efforts. This tendency can show up in a variety of spheres of life, including career pursuits and physical exercise regimens. In the context of fitness, it's important to recognize that the body might become accustomed to a particular training regimen and eventually produce fewer benefits when discussing plateaus. People ought to think about mixing up their routines to get around this. To shock the body into reacting favorably, this could entail trying a new fitness class, stepping up the intensity, or switching up the types of exercises.

Furthermore, plateaus are frequently accompanied by psychological difficulties because people may feel discouraged and tempted to give up on their fitness objectives. Reevaluating both short- and long-term goals, maintaining focus, and acknowledging non-scale successes is crucial. Motivation can be sustained by acknowledging that plateaus are a normal part of any journey and setting reasonable expectations.

Seeking help from a fitness group or a professional trainer can also provide vital insights and encouragement during these hard periods.

DEALING WITH CRAVINGS

Cravings are a ubiquitous difficulty when it comes to keeping a good diet, and they may weaken even the most diligent persons. Understanding the fundamental reasons for cravings is key to effective management. Cravings often result from a mix of physiological and psychological causes, such as dietary deficits, emotional stress, or conditioned responses to certain stimuli. Identifying these triggers is the first step towards establishing solutions to deal with cravings.

One effective technique is to focus on nutrient-dense foods that satisfy the body's nutritional needs. Ensuring a balanced diet that includes a variety of macronutrients and micronutrients can help reduce cravings linked to nutrient deficiencies. Additionally, practicing mindfulness and recognizing emotional triggers can aid in breaking the cycle of emotional eating. Incorporating healthier alternatives for indulgent cravings, such as choosing dark chocolate over sugary treats, allows for a more balanced approach without completely depriving oneself.

Developing a support system can also be instrumental in managing cravings. Sharing challenges and successes with friends, family, or a support group can provide accountability and encouragement during moments of temptation. Finally, establishing a realistic and sustainable approach to dieting, rather than adhering to extreme restrictions, can contribute to a healthier relationship with food and reduce the likelihood of succumbing to cravings.

ADJUSTING THE DIET FOR CHILDREN

Adapting a child's diet to ensure optimal nutrition is a concern for many parents.

One common challenge is striking the right balance between providing a variety of nutrients essential for growth and development while accommodating a child's preferences. Encouraging healthy eating habits early in life is crucial, and parents often face resistance from children who may prefer processed or sugary foods.

To address this challenge, parents can involve children in the meal planning and preparation process. Allowing them to make choices within healthy options can empower children and increase their interest in nutritious foods. Creating a positive and enjoyable eating environment, such as family meals, can also contribute to better dietary habits.

Limiting access to sugary snacks and promoting the consumption of whole foods, fruits, and vegetables can establish a foundation for a balanced diet.

Moreover, understanding individual nutritional needs based on age and activity level is essential for adjusting a child's diet. Regular communication with pediatricians or nutritionists can provide valuable guidance on specific dietary requirements for different developmental stages.